MORNING CUNNILINGUS

*How To Wake Your Partner Up
With Oral Sex*

Dr. Steve Ross David

0

TABLE OF CONTENT

INTRODUCTION

Being awakened with oral sex is a typical dream, however, while it could sound hot, there's a great deal to consider before you make it a reality. It's dependably essential to talk about limits with your accomplice, yet in this present circumstance, it's fundamental.

This book contains the perspective on 104 men and ladies on morning sex: why they like it, why they could do without it and what makes it unbelievable.

Regardless of whether you right now battle to climax during sex or while stroking off, this book will likewise work for you.

Also, the best part is that you don't have to do anything unusual or awkward to begin having the best climaxes and sex of your life.

STEP BY STEP INSTRUCTIONS TO AWAKEN YOUR PARTNER WITH ORAL SEX

While having a go at something new or satisfying an accomplice's dream, openness is of the utmost importance. "Many couples have unequivocal and understood arrangements about unambiguous exercises. For example, many couples don't need assent while giving each other a kiss or an embrace, while they will ask each other for a back rub or sex." to make this dream a reality, you can "totally" pull out all the stops — yet discuss it first.

While examining this dream with your accomplice, incorporate some sharing around limits, as, 'Do you believe I should shock you with awaken oral, or would you favor we prepare of time?' 'Is there daily that turns out better for you, similar to Saturday morning?' 'Is there anything you know about that would keep you from partaking in this amazement?'" Become point by point about facilitated activities, but think further, too.

"Be interested about why this dream turns your accomplice on.

In particular, examine what "being awakened with oral sex" signifies — does your accomplice need to be conscious however languid before oral starts? Is it true or not that they are fine on the off chance that they're somewhere down in a REM cycle? Perhaps they might want to be half-conscious? Discuss how they'd like sex to work out: would they like in the first place foreplay, or would they like to go directly to oral? Discuss it so that when you start, you understand what your accomplice is and isn't happy with.

On the off chance that your accomplice isn't into being awakened with oral sex (or awakening you with oral sex), perhaps you can track down one more method for integrating what you see as so hot about this thought. For instance, perhaps you choose to have oral sex when you're both alert, yet before you've gotten up and had your morning espresso. Or on the other hand perhaps you choose to integrate the situation into pretend.

"Dreams are thoughts that stir us and give us joy when we ponder them. Wants are things we really need to do," says Master. "In some cases a dream turns into a longing and the experience is brilliant. In any case, now and again dreams that significantly turn us on don't feel quite a bit better when we act them out. Frequently, this can be cured with clear correspondence between accomplices, delicate criticism, and practice."

Notwithstanding, this isn't generally the situation. A few dreams are improved left as private considering or filthy talk with an accomplice. "Since there are a few things that give us more joy when we ponder them instead of encountering them. Realizing the distinction will assist you with boosting your true capacity for encountering joy and association."

On the off chance that you and your accomplice choose to put it all on the line, this is what to do: begin slow. In the event that you're giving a sensual caress, center around the head first before profound throating. Assuming that you're eating somebody out, begin by licking their clit gradually. Focus on your accomplice and let their responses be your aide.

Remember that assent can continuously be removed, so assuming you start awakening your collaborate with oral and they don't appear into it, stop right away and check in with them. Then again, on the off chance that your accomplice is groaning and telling you not to stop, tune in and appreciate; a large portion of us view our accomplice's sex sounds as really hot, all things considered.

11 Methods for having Better Morning Sex.

Ok, morning sex. Some thoroughly stay away from it, others basically love it. In the event that you're not an ascent and-drudgery (in a real sense) sort of individual, we're trusting you can gain proficiency with a specialist tip or two here that will adjust your perspective. What's more, assuming you're about awaken sex, I have hot exhortation from stars that will take your AM normal to a higher level.

Be that as it may, before you get everything rolling — for what reason do such countless docs and specialists depend on an early meeting between the sheets? Is it actually the best opportunity to engage in sexual relations, as so many case? It's basic. "The most amazing part of morning sex is that you are revived and free."

"Unwinding is the groundwork of excitement and in the first part of the day prior to the buzzing about of your day is an ideal chance to get provocative with your accomplice."

"Testosterone levels are higher in the first part of the day prompting expanded sexual longing." Underneath are morning sex benefits as well as certain ideas for the best sexual positions.

1. Joy yourself first.

"Mornings start deferred for a considerable number of individuals so morning sex should not be unreasonably terrifying or athletic."

"Stir up your own blazes via stroking yourself to energy, then begin dealing with delicate touches and delicate kisses to your accomplice's body."

What's more, when things heat up with your accomplice, don't feel like you want to make a direct route to the restroom to clean your teeth: "On the off chance that you have an inclination that sex may be straightaway, take a speedy taste of water to bring some relief."

2. Lurk into some hot oral.

On the off chance that day to day sex is an objective for yourself as well as your accomplice, consider alternating pleasuring one another. "A minuscule measure of foreplay in the initial segment of the day has a wonderful effect."

"Oral sex is generally a fast and serene method for getting somebody off in the first part of the day, and an ideal method for extinguishing wants in a fantastic state."

3. Or on the other hand go for that 69.

"69 is an incredible situation for morning sex since you don't need to stress over morning breath or having a hesitant outlook on what you look like." "You can utilize your hands and mouth to invigorate your accomplice's body and investigate sucking, licking, stroking, and pleasuring your collaborate with your mouth and hands." Hello, you must clean your teeth after you get up at any rate, so you should do it before you even outfit for the afternoon.

4. Express welcome to shower foreplay.

In a rush? Then, at that point, wrench up your shower and kill two birds with one...nozzle. "Sex in the shower can stir you and be an extraordinary technique for starting your day."

On the whole, attempt this: "Begin with washed each other up and feeling the sensations as the water hits your body. Kiss and stroke your accomplice and investigate various types of touch and excitement." Recollect, shower sex can come in many structures. You can decide available feeling or shared masturbation to make things hot while you bubbles up.

5. Then, at that point, enjoy some all out shower sex.

Most importantly, you will need lube on the off chance that you are participating in shower sex that includes entrance, whether it's with a penis or a sex toy. Why? "In spite of the fact that it might appear to be unreasonable, all possible endeavors at shower sex ought to incorporate lube. The wealth of water washes away normal grease, which can have a drying impact and make entrance self-conscious."

Presently, onto the tomfoolery stuff: "A night shower could permit additional opportunity to pull off those more brave positions, however in the early hours keep them protected and basic. Get going remaining with your hands squeezed against the shower wall and your legs marginally spread, and have your accomplice enter you from behind." As you anchor yourself with your hands established on the wall, this will let loose your accomplice's hands to meander all around your body.

6. Attempt some spooning.

Of course, you can't kiss here. Be that as it may, assuming morning breath is a worry, swing this nevertheless feel personally associated with your accomplice. "In the event that you rest in the spoon position, essentially press those spoons together a piece nearer." In the event that you're not a prompt riser lover, think about this: "Contributing energy close to one another and partaking in sex can convey oxytocin — the compound at risk for vibes of affiliation and prosperity."

7. Get off in cowgirl.

"Instead of the spooning position, cowgirl could have all the earmarks of being a lot of work," "Yet considering the way that it's one of the most orgasmic positions for women, and you're getting up exactly on schedule to complete the thing in any event, ought to get the most incentive for your cash." With your accomplice on their back and you holding the rules up top, you'll oversee profundity and speed — so you can focus in on what feels best for you.

"Rather than bouncing everywhere (which, might we at any point be genuine, it's probable too early for), have a go at shaking all over or turning your hips."

Concerning flooding your body with that large number of feel-great chemicals? That is a damn decent sans java morning shock we can get behind.

8. Center around more modest demonstrations of touch.

It's the morning. You're actually drained. Your grimy talk jargon may not be going full bore and your appendages might be similarly close. Focus on minuscule actual blessings for your S/O — regardless of whether it's not out and out sex — and your psyche and body will be happy you did. Turns out there are a great deal of advantages to peaking in the AM.

"In the event that you have an unpleasant day coming up, your body will begin to see its cortisol levels (also called 'the pressure chemical') ascent," the sex and relationship. "Regardless, did you had in any event a few thought that a make-out and settle close to the start of the day can adjust this? At the point when you kiss and snuggle, nerve motivations go through the skin and your fringe nerves to go up the spine to the cerebrum, where they invigorate the arrival of oxytocin (the 'nestle chemical'), as well as serotonin and dopamine (the 'cheerful chemicals'). Therefore, you feel not so much pushed but rather more horny."

To heighten these sentiments, direct your accomplice to kiss your erogenous zones like your ears, neck, or "whether you feel the most sensation, as this will divert you from your forthcoming day considerably more so."

9. Add some toys.

Let a battery-fueled joy or dildo accomplish some work when you're at your groggiest. "Flavor your mornings up by adding sex toys to your initial morning happiness," it is recommended for ladies to utilize clit triggers and rooster rings, particularly assuming your accomplice is somebody who has issues remaining or getting hard toward the beginning of the day. "Sex toys can be an unprecedented technique for getting you past the edge towards topping."

10. Treat your accomplice to a back rub.

"There isn't anything more unwinding than getting up in the first part of the day, getting a sexy back rub, and afterward getting laid." "What better method for beginning your day than that?"

Green prescribes evaluating various oils to see which you like best and to trade among you and your accomplice every morning who will be giving/getting the back rub. Doing light accomplice extending is one more decent choice to iron out every one of the wrinkles, as well. sex positions like the butterfly, libra, ballet dancer, and the canyon to take your extending up a level to new sexual levels.

11. Contemplate sex the prior night.

Master offers this guidance to prime yourself for heavenly sex in the A.M. "Contemplating sex the earlier night is one of the most exceptional approaches to setting up your mind for sex in the initial segment of the day." "While it doesn't need to be the final thing you consider before you nod off, it merits fantasizing about the next morning as it could prompt you having a sex dream, thusly, making you much hornier in the first part of the day."

Discussing preparing, it's smart to have lube convenient for morning sex, as certain ladies experience grease issues in the first part of the day. "Numerous people acknowledge that lube is totally used by individuals who experience the evil impacts of dryness during sex, but this verifiably isn't correct and conveys a lot of benefits to the room. As far as one might be concerned, it can improve delight by causing various situations like a warming or cooling impact any place it's applied." "Past examinations have shown that lube makes it half simpler for everybody to climax." On that note, time to fantasize about tomorrow first thing as you float off to Lala land.

TOP TIPS FOR THE BEST MORNING SEX AS AFFIRMED BY MEN AND LADIES

The following are the assessments of people on why morning sex is inconceivable. The perspectives and encounters of 35 men on having incredible morning sex and obviously, criticism from 19 individuals who could do without morning sex.

50 Ladies Make sense of Why Morning Sex Is Mind blowing

Underneath you are criticisms from 50 ladies on why they like morning sex and the tips they use to make it incredible:

1.   It's the most ideal way to awaken. A hard rooster between my butt cheeks, becoming more enthusiastically and longer as he tenderly gets me

up with morning kisses!! It just got the day going with the best grin and mind-set.

2.   It's close and unconstrained. It's a pleasant method for brightening up your penis massage abilities. Likewise causes me to feel pretty and that I am still visually captivating to him when I awaken.

3.   It's fantastic to awaken my collaborate with a remarkable sensual caress!

4.   I love morning sex, particularly on vacation. You have the most energy and you can return to rest assuming you need after it. I love feeling sleepy and get turned on. Additionally, his penis is more diligently toward the beginning of the day, it's faster and more enthusiastic.

5.   I think morning sex is generally excellent on the grounds that there isn't much to plan for- simple access and both loose and invigorated from resting.

6.   The serenity and energy.

7.   For me, it's a perspective. At the point when the morning begins with joy then there is delight the entire day. I feel loose, fulfilled and sure.

8.   Spooning and grating against a hard chicken, hands stroking my body, neck kisses, and delicate murmurs letting me know how lovely I turn when I wake upward. The closeness and close association it makes when still not appropriately conscious and my normal magnificence is wanted.

9.   Morning sex generally bests any remaining seasons of day for sex. The man's moxie is most noteworthy between 6 am and 9 am. I don't know why it feels such a great deal better for me toward the beginning of the day. Perhaps on the grounds that his sex drive makes his craving pinnacle and it's as a rule before the youngsters are conscious.

10.   Just awakening close to somebody you love and engaging in sexual relations first thing in the AM is perfect.

11.   Waking dependent upon him going down on me. Causes you to feel like you are the principal thing he needs.

12.   The sensation is such a great deal better in the event that you start when you're scarcely conscious and your brain is a fresh start.

13.   When it begins sweet and cherishing.

14.   I LOVE morning sex, it's my number one! Awakening horny and extremely drowsy to turn over to an exposed body is the absolute best! Going slowly in a lethargic state to appreciate foreplay and satisfy each other is extremely fulfilling. Likewise beginning your day with a climax is entirely pleasurable.

15.   When we have the entire day to our selves return up make espresso and come once again to bed I feel more ready and loose without anything to do. There is additional opportunity for foreplay and a more profound association. We attempt various points and find what feels better.

16.   It's very nearly a continuation of the prior night and sets one up for the afternoon.

17.   We wake up loaded up with sexual fervor, sort of tired, and our hair is chaotic, and the elevating morning light in the room improves it than night sex.

18.   I am more stirred first thing, all around rested, and all set.

19.   He awakens me by contacting me or going down on me and we have intercourse until we both peak. Then we snuggle and fall back to rest.

20.   I love realizing that I'm the first thing he needs in quite a while day, that his previously thought or feeling is the craving to accompany me. The most fulfilling morning sex is generally following an evening of extraordinary, harsher energy. Better, gentler, more slow morning sex that broadens the delight and arrives at the opposite finish of my range is awesome.

21.   I like all morning sex. It is the point at which I'm the most loose so climaxes are more straightforward for me.

22.   He can go much harder and longer.

It is so great to 23.   morning butt-centric sex. I love it. I don't why however my butthole feels so loosened up in the first part of the day and I'm somewhat horny when I see my man lying bare close to me. I lean toward doing butt-centric in the mornings.

24.   I love when my accomplice tenderly kisses me to awaken me and afterward licks my clit until I'm going to peak and afterward screws me.

25.   I just normally awaken horny.

26.   The sluggish liveliness.

27.   'Cause I'm on top and in charge.

28.   When I'm still sleeping and he slides directly into me and awakens me!

29.   When you awaken horny, your sexual longings are 10x more serious. Each touch resembles a rush.

30.   Who requirements caffeine when there is sex?

31.   I consistently feel the most weak in the first part of the day and I like to be overwhelmed in the room.

32.   The best morning sex I've had is the point at which I can't rest around evening time and I'm up really early. A decent pussy eating or a pleasant fuck generally encourages me.

33.   Silent spooning fixes a headache.

34.   It's so warm and wet in the first part of the day.

35.   It's pleasurable in light of the fact that I'm enamored with that individual and there's nothing better in this world than to detect him, us, before the day starts.

36.   Love morning sex. Normally, the person is feeling destitute and delicate.

37.   Waking up close to your darling inclination a staggering inclination to satisfy him in any capacity conceivable.

38.   The best morning sex is extraordinary and enthusiastic and leaves the two players totally

thrilled about one another until the end of the day. Most effective way to begin the day!

39.   Usually, my accomplice starts off ahead of schedule for work, so my main goal is to keep him in the bed as long as I can, so we play this little game... In the event that he winds up behind schedule for work, I won!

40.   I'm extremely delicate in the first part of the day, it resembles my clit and vagina are as of now pre-excited. Morning sex is a major treat.

41.   Because it in a real sense interfaces dreams to the real world.

42.   When we don't need to hurry to work... And we both get muddled.

43.   Morning sex with my accomplice is fun since he actually behaves like hes making an effort not to start it however I can feel him getting hard against my butt. Also, we typically bother each other until we start really getting into it.

44.   Drowsy drowsy sex is suggestive.

45.   Morning sex, more loose, full bladder I think that prompting extraordinary climaxes.

46.   I love morning sex! The squirms and stretches and professing to in any case be sleeping is consistently fun.

47.   My accomplice likes to nestle in the early morning hours, which obviously fires up my motor a piece when he gets gushy. He some of the time begins a stimulate war which gets my adrenaline rolling, and the best sex is the point at which you are entirely stirred with an increase in adrenaline.

48.   It was ideal to see my man's demeanors and so that him could see mine and he can see my body more with the daylight coming in. It caused us to feel truly associated with one another.

49.   Because I'm enamored with him each time we talk or I see him I in a split second feel horny.

50.   I'm in every case truly turned on toward the beginning of the day, I love it when we don't talk yet we understand what we need.

35 Men Discuss Why Morning Sex Is So Charming

The following are the accommodation from 35 men:

1.   Morning head is incredible on the grounds that it's not normal.

2.   It's like awakening and working out while still half-bewildered and sleeping.

3.   When she's actually splashing from the prior night.

4.   My accomplice feels the horniest promptly toward the beginning of the day.

5.   It's generally more erotic, milder, and charmingly unusual.

6.   It takes more time to cum and furthermore my accomplice can cum on different occasions.

7.   In the morning she is new, you are new, and the sex is an effective method for beginning a day.

8.   When I awaken is the point at which I'm the horniest.

9.   It gives you complete closeness before the stressors of the day.

10.   Because its heartfelt.

11.   When I'm in a profound rest and I wake up with my hands playing with my young lady's wet pussy. The best sex is morning sex gives over.

12.   The immediacy, all things considered, is the best piece. I don't view it has as too lengthy, only 3 or 4 minutes and completely fine's.

13.   I love morning sex; an incredible method for beginning the day. It gets the blood siphoning. It's generally quicker on the grounds that we need to get to work. Everything is regular, my woman is delicate, flexible and I love beginning her day feeling unique.

14.   Because my dick is now hard and she doesn't have the foggiest idea about its coming.

15.   When you awaken following some serious time sex and its stone hard and all set once more. It's basic.

16.   Morning sex is generally an astonishing method for beginning the day in addition to she appeared to have less restraints.

17.   When I awaken adjacent to her and simply have her everything to myself, it is extremely fulfilling. Love when I'm inside her, and time doesn't make any difference.

18.   When she begins the day riding me and my chicken is so difficult, in the first place, we scarcely need to practice after that. Revived and prepared for the showers! No better chance to tell her the amount you love her.

19.   Sleepy, warm, agreeable, profound association, feeling adored, engaging.

20.   It is extremely extraordinary and natural. We awaken, look, at one another, and recently began screwing. It happens frequently particularly when we're holiday.

21.   The best morning sex is the point at which my significant other awakens me with a hand work and continues to ride me when I turned out to be hard. It's extraordinary in light of the fact

that my brain is clear and to see her body first thing is amazing!

22. All morning sex is great. It's good to awaken close to your accomplice when you are both bare and nestle up close to her and just tenderly begin running your hand once again her and gradually begin to feel her body get energized. Her areolas get hard, her pussy gets wet. She moves to a position where I can contact her bosoms all the more effectively and she opens her legs so I can play with her pussy...

23. The most fulfilling morning sex is following an evening of sex. A few times, after an extreme night of a few rounds of sex, awakening in a nestling position, and it's not difficult to go one more round as though a continuation of what happened only a couple of hours prior. Then, at that point, return to rest for an hour or so prior to beginning the day.

24. Her pussy feels more sultry.

25. The explanation morning sex is extremely fulfilling is that the body and brain had a few rest

and the degree of strain in the sensory system is exceptionally low. This makes the body ingest and appreciate sex much better and more profound than when the body and brain are loaded with strain from every one of the exercises and feelings from an entire day's occasions.

26. Feeling of closeness and acknowledgment (she's there and accessible for anything).

27. Waking up with my sweetheart close to me in the entirety of her brilliance, looking provocative as damnation and simply sliding on top of me and taking me somewhere inside.

28. To beginning the day with your first love so exotically makes the remainder of the day better.

29. Shower sex is perfect in the first part of the day — and water sports.

30. When I'm revived from a decent night's rest during which I fantasized engaging in sexual relations.

31. The surge of completing to some degree rapidly and knowing that assuming I pull her hair

and make her chaotic, it very well may be seen by her associates was stimulating.

32.   The best morning sex is that tired, gropey, sluggish fuck. Something about laying there, interlaced, gradually fucking without saying a lot of feels so private. At the point when we engage in sexual relations around evening time it's not unexpected a huge creation. Toys, underwear, lube, sexual dreams, and so on yet morning sex feels more... cuddly perhaps? Really adoring and erotic? I love it for truly associating on a profound level with my better half.

33.   I love it when a young lady awakens me since she needs to have intercourse. She begins contacting me, contacting my dick, and before I'm even truly alert she has that dick in her mouth preparing it hard and. It makes me wild.

34.   Before I moved in with my accomplice, I would drive consistently to her home, we would be up around 50% of the late evening engaging in sexual relations, then, at that point, get up in the

first part of the day for one more round, she's staggering.

35. I value awakening close to my significant other each day however sex is only the good to beat all. No expectation, mulling over everything... Just normally occurs and is wonderful. Most effective way to begin the day without a doubt.

19 INDIVIDUALS MAKE SENSE OF HOW MORNING SEX CAN BE UNINSPIRING

Obviously, not every person likes morning sex, so you ought to likewise realize the reason why certain individuals think that it is unenjoyable:

1.   During morning sex you can't kiss as the morning inhale might be frightful.

2.   When I am fretted over being working at a specific time.

3.   If I feel gross from perspiring in the evening (from being too warm in the late spring for instance), it's difficult to get into it.

4.   Monthly cycle cramps prior to getting an opportunity to take Tylenol or model. Back torment. Or on the other hand the kids getting up during morning sex. Side note: Strong ways to have incredible sex on your period.

5. Sometimes it takes more time to truly get into it in the event that you're not prepared to awaken.

6. If they aren't an early riser and wake up testy. Despite the fact that sex can now and again change that.

7. When it resembles a fast in and out and he's surging out the way to leave. Causes you kind of to feel objectified.

8. Sometimes there will be a slight unwanted fragrance from sex the prior night. I truly wouldn't fret since I realize I'm smelling our lovemaking.

9. If I'm truly sluggish being in the mood is difficult.

10. If my accomplice is simply making a halfhearted effort/isn't actually into it.

11. When I'm not in that frame of mind and he is attempting to get me into it. Particularly on the off chance that I was worn out from the prior night.

12.   If he needs butt-centric and I haven't crapped.

13.   If I'm not completely alert and he hasn't gotten some margin to turn me on. Then, at that point, it's awkward. Or on the other hand in the event that he rips the sheets off me and I get cold.

14.   Sometimes I don't have morning wood and a significant chunk of time must pass.

15.   It differs from one accomplice to another, the way things are drawn nearer and quietly mentioning it. On the off chance that I'm not willing, kindly don't drive it. Yet, not being prepared isn't exactly the same thing as not being willing.

16.   Just that my psyche is in 6 different bearings. In this way, it's difficult for me to get truly into it, not to mention finish.

17.   The pee smell and taste on the off chance that an accomplice needs oral sex.

18.   When my bladder is full and I haven't peed.

19.   When I get my period.

The Miscreants View On Morning Sex

There are a lot of pluses to having intercourse in the first part of the day.

1.   You get the day going feeling great.

2.   You'll convey that "after sex" sparkle with you to work or school!

3.   No one needs to rest in the wet spot.

4.   It can replace your morning exercise.

5.   Sunlight floating through the shades can be very heartfelt.

6.   You're not pondering the rest you're passing up on the grounds that you're now very much refreshed!

7.   You don't need to stress over wrinkling garments you should wear once more.

8.   There's compelling reason need to stress over putting your best self forward first thing.

9.   Oxytocin, which is delivered during sex and nestling, assists you with feeling near your man the entire day.

10.   Morning sex three times each week might try and diminish chance of coronary failures! Source.

11.   The expansion in testosterone men experience in the first part of the day might assist him with enduring longer.

There's no really great explanations for why morning sex is amazing. That languid inclination can cause the entire thing to appear to be really strange, and you may be more carnal before your mind kicks into a more "human" mode. While you could regularly go after some espresso, think about morning sex, all things being equal.

Sex in the first part of the day may be a decent choice in the event that you much of the time wind up falling asleep around evening time before you and your man get an opportunity to strip each other down. Furthermore, assuming you truly do end up carving out opportunity to waste time at least a few times during the day? Then, at that point, good luck with that! So set your alert 30 minutes to an hour sooner. You don't need to let your man in on what's happening assuming you realize he'll be down for morning sex!

Which infers whether or not it's OK to awaken your accomplice - or be awakened - with sex. It tends to be hot to be stirred from fantasy land since somebody's slipping hands inside your underwear, grabbing your bosoms or fingering you, however it's not a great fit for everybody. On the off chance that this is the sort of thing you're available to, let your man know in advance. Furthermore, assuming that you'd prefer get rest for your huge show, let him know, as well.

Make a point to find out where he remains on the issue since, as opposed to mainstream thinking, all men don't need sex constantly! Assent is significant, regardless of whether you've previously had intercourse one or multiple times, regardless of whether you're in a serious relationship. It's so significant, we can't discuss things, for example, BDSM or tipsy sex without referencing it!

HOW TO MAKE MORNING SEX GREAT?

1. Tell Him You Need It

One method for telling your man you're OK is by resting without clothing - or without anything by any means. There are different advantages to resting exposed, as well. Regardless of whether you end up having intercourse, you'll feel pretty magnificent resting exposed.

You can likewise energize him by squeezing your body facing him. What lady hasn't exploited spooning to urge her man to get in that frame of mind? Assuming you find that dozing exposed gets you horny, you might begin by stroking off. When your man is stir by it - a couple of key groans can help - he can participate. Or then again perhaps you'll simply adhere to common masturbation. It very well may be unbelievably hot!

2. Keep Condoms Close by

Many individuals keep condoms or different sorts of contraception promptly accessible in the end table cabinet. It's particularly essential to make sure to utilize anti-conception medication when you could not completely be alert. Contraception, for example, the stomach, Nuva ring or wipe can be embedded beforehand,which may be valuable when you're in the state of mind for morning sex.

3. Attempt It Outside

On the off chance that you live where the mornings are warm, sneak outside for a quick in and out on your deck furniture or take a stab at having intercourse in your sun room. As the sun rises, you'll get an incredible view. It'll feel perfect, as well. On the off chance that there's a gamble of being gotten, you could appreciate it considerably more! Be that as it may, you must be cautious while having intercourse outside.

4. Serve It With Breakfast

This one works when you're the person who ordinarily awakens first, yet trying out taking care of him toward the beginning of the day on the off chance that that is not typically your everyday practice as can show him the amount you care about his pleasure. You can eat began, and when you let him in on it's served, be exposed when he goes into the room. Play it safe. A cover shields sensitive skin from oil splatters. What's more, you might not have any desire to make anything hot by any means on the off chance that it will get cold as you play around.

Something senseless like holding doughnuts over your areolas can show that's prepared for the taking. You can likewise involve the counter or table as a prop during your lovemaking meeting. The Consuming Man position is perfect for this. Also, you can hang over the counter for back passage or butt-centric sex positions.

5. Shock Ride Him

Obviously, numerous men have boo boos in the first part of the day because of elevated degrees of testosterone and expanded blood stream during rest, which makes morning an ideal opportunity to ride him. A lot of men couldn't want anything more than to get up to a morning shock like this.

Think about switch cowgirl, as well. This position assists with managing that morning breath issue. Besides, you get an alternate point and you have some control over the profundity and speed of pushing. It's reasonable assuming that you feel reluctant with regards to being on top during sex.

6. Wake Him Up with Oral Sex

One more method for ensuring your man awakens blissful is to energize him from sleep with your mouth on his rooster. Obviously, awakening to your man moving between your legs is comparably great, so you can drop a couple of clues that you might want to awaken to this.

Additionally, in the event that you're a person understanding this, you might need to think about awakening your female join forces with oral sex, as such a greater part of ladies like getting oral sex.

7. Keep it Loose with Spooning

Morning sex is marvelous on the grounds that it's frequently 'tired' and languid, and you don't have to do any kind of aerobatic in light of the fact that you're not as yet completely alert. This is one justification for why spooning is a particularly decent position. You can be near your accomplice, and both of you can invigorate your clitoris, yet you can keep the speed loose. Furthermore, you don't need to manage morning breath, which can be a mind-set executioner!

8. Do It in the Shower

Another choice is to have intercourse in the first part of the day while you're in the shower. Shower can be unimaginably hot when done well. Ensure there's no way of slipping, which could prompt injury. On the off chance that you need, add a waterproof toy, and a lot of silicone-based lube (since water isn't great for your normal oil), you're all set.

CONCLUSION

Ideally these ideas provide you with certain thoughts of your own, whether you're new to engaging in sexual relations in the first part of the day or you're an accomplished ace. In the event that it's something you don't regularly do, your person may be open to your advances. Or on the other hand you could understand it simply doesn't function admirably with your timetable, and that is OK, as well. There's nobody way or ideal opportunity for you to engage in sexual relations, which is the reason testing is such a lot of tomfoolery!

Regardless of whether you presently battle to climax during sex or while jerking off, this book will likewise work for you.

Also, the best part is that you don't have to do anything odd or awkward to begin having the best climaxes and sex of your life.